Essential Oils: The Complete Guide

Essential Oils Guide for Beginners, Aromatherapy & Weight Loss.

Free Bonus Book: 50 DIY Essential Oils Recipes Available Inside.

By Coral James

Introduction

Have you ever struggled with doctors? Have you found that they deem some things "un-diagnosable" or that they treat symptoms individually until they figure out the actual cause or just alleviate the symptoms temporarily? Western medicine is inherently flawed in that it focuses on the symptoms and works from the stand point of testing for everything until only one possible cause is left. It does not focus on the entire body or the person. Instead it utilizes a medical history chart and offers medications that often cause more permanent harm to the body than good. Medications are also prescribed for a specific symptom and not necessarily an entire illness. As you target one symptom you may not be targeting the cause of the symptom. Aromatherapy does not do that. It offers a natural way to reduce stress and lose weight in a way that embodies your mind, body, and spirit. Utilizing all of these concepts it restores and adjusts the balance inside your body in a very holistic manner. It allows you to self-regulate, self-repair, and maintain harmony between your body and nature.

Chapter One: Understanding Aromatherapy

Aromatherapy is really the therapeutic use of essential oils which are taken from plants. Studies indicate that aromatherapy brings with it multiple health benefits including relief from stress and anxiety, and an improved quality of life particularly for people who suffer from chronic health conditions brought about by weight gain from stress. The essential oils that are used in aromatherapy are generally extracted from different parts of plants and then distilled. The concentrated oils can be applied directly to the skin through bath salts, lotions, soaps or massages, or they can be inhaled directly and indirectly through the burning of candles and incense. Aromatherapy works by stimulating the smell receptors in your nose which then send messages throughout your nervous system to your limbic system where your emotions are controlled.

Aromatherapy

You can take advantage of key scents and flavors integrated into everyday items such as body lotion, candles, oils, incense, shower gels, hand soaps, and more. You can integrate aromatherapy into a professional massage or in your home. Aromatherapy can enhance your mood and give you an improved feeling of well-being. If you expose yourself to essential aromatherapy oils during a massage, for example, you improve your blood and circulation which can reduce your blood pressure, something which is often heightened by extreme weight gain or stress. Essential oils can help to balance the hormone production inside of your endocrine system. They can strengthen your immune system by helping to kill off bacterial fungal infections as well as viruses. They can improve digestion, something that often is hindered by excessive stress or weight gain. Aromatherapy can reduce pain and can encourage restful sleep, something which is particularly important for reducing weight and stress.

How it Works

People respond on an emotional level to their sense of smell stronger than they do to any of the other five senses. One single aroma can trigger a forgotten memory. One single aroma can remind you of a calmer time and alleviate all stress. The limbic system is the part of the brain which is associated with memory and smell. The olfactory nerves inside of your nasal cavity respond to the aromas associated with aromatherapy. This information is then sent up to the limbic system where it connects with the pituitary gland in the hypothalamus, areas of the brain which govern the hormonal systems. Certain aromas can trigger a plethora of chemical reactions inside your body. They can release specific chemicals which can relax, stimulate or create a general feeling of health and well-being. Aromatherapy can energize you and lift you up, help you to maintain healthy joints and muscles, alleviate stress, revive your mind and body, and create a tranquil ambience.

The History of Aromatherapy

Aromatherapy dates to prehistoric times. Juniper berries were used to add flavor to food and were also used as an antiseptic. Evidence indicates that civilizations throughout the centuries have used plants and herbs for cosmetic, culinary, and medicinal purposes. The Egyptians used plant oils during the process of mummification. Frankincense has been located in Egyptian tombs. Multiple fragrance oils were used for cosmetics as well as for rituals. Egyptian incense often included fragrant oils such as lemongrass, juniper, cardamom, and frankincense. Frankincense was so highly regarded that in many cases it was revered as more valuable than gold. The ancient Greeks learned some of their knowledge on the use of plants in medicine from the Egyptians. Greek physicians used chamomile to reduce fevers and integrated this plant into daily massages to improve health. Other aromatic herbs were also used in massages to reduce complaints of physical ailments. During the medieval period Persian physicians discovered the process of distillation which contributed a great deal to the use of essential oils not only in massages but in fragrant public baths. It became commonplace to integrate essential oils into Roman culture through the use of public bath houses. In China and India the use of plants and herbs for medicinal purposes is long and thorough. Sandalwood was used by Chinese physicians to treat things such as cholera. Clover buds were kept in the mouth in order to ease bad breath. The Emperor's book of internal medicine is still used today, and contains treatments for the body, spirit, and mind. In India the use of sandalwood was used as an exorcism right and to heal wounds. Plants were used to treat the ailments of knights returning from their crusades. They were used to treat skin conditions and respiratory conditions as well as to protect against infection. Essential oils was classed as the medicine of the people, and the women of each household were responsible for making these home remedies for their families.

It was in the 18th century that apothecaries began to add essential oils to their list of products. The healing properties of lavender oil was actually discovered by mistake when a french chemist burnt his hand on lavender oil and discovered the healing properties. Essential oils were used in military hospitals during the First World War, the findings of which were published in a scientific research paper in the year 1928. It was at this point that the term aromatherapy was first used.

Aromatherapy as a form of therapy was continually researched during the Indochina war and around the world massage treatments began to integrate essential oils. Soon after, the use of aromatherapy became a widely accepted international therapy.

Chapter Two: Your Mind, Body, and Spirit

Your Mind

Aromatherapy is a catalyst for change in your mind, body and spirit. Essential oils stimulate the area of your brain which affect emotions. The oil molecules are absorbed through the nose and sent through the nervous system. Once they pass through the nervous system they return to the limbic system where pleasure and emotions are perceived and where your memories are stored. When your limbic system is stimulated it releases chemicals which have an effect on the central nervous system. These chemicals include endorphins which reduce pain and serotonin which counteracts anxiety. Inhaling essential oils can help to give an emotional balance. Being in an emotionally balanced state brings with it a therapeutic effect for other physical problems including stress and weight gain. You can enhance your mental well-being through the direct inhalation of essential oils or the diffusion of essential oils. You can inhale the oils directly if you need immediate relief. For example, if you are stressed and need to relax you can apply drops of chamomile oil onto a handkerchief and hold it under your nose. Because of the volatile nature of essential oils they will very quickly diffuse into the air. An aromatherapy lamp has a small basin in which the essential oils and water are mixed and the scent is diffused. This basin is warmed from underneath by a candle. Some diffusing oils like sandalwood, chamomile, and rose can help you to feel more at ease when you are particularly stressed. If you are feeling lethargic and need a lift you can use peppermint, basil, or lemon.

Your Body

Essential oils can be quickly absorbed through your skin via hair follicles. Essential oils enter the glands and mingle with your skin. These chemical properties can be balancing, cleansing, or toning. Essential oils provide an aesthetic dimension to the healing effects of a facial steam, a bath, a compress, or massage therapy. Because they are heavily concentrated, essential oils have to be diluted which means they often compose 2 to 3% of a blend of vegetable oils like sweet almond oil. This is the normal percentage you will find in body care products. For example just a few drops of grapefruit oil added to a warm bath can help to reduce stress. The largest organ of the body is the skin. And the state in which your skin is serves as a reflection of your inner state of well-being. That is why it is imperative to take care of your skin through the use of aromatherapy. Certain oils are particularly suited to benefit your skin. Lavender oil, for example, will tone, balance, cleanse and deodorize your skin. It will literally wash away the stress and the unhealthy visible side effects of weight gain. Lavender is also relatively safe in a higher dilution, upwards of 20%. Lavender oil can replenish dry skin and soothe the body.

Your spirit

The scent from an oil diffuser can waft around your room like a mysterious presence, helping meditation and penetrating deeply into your lungs to help regulate your breath. Diffusing oils such as frankincense can help to carry you from a stressful work day into a spiritual journey of relaxation at home. Essential oils bring with them positive effects on every level of your being. Each oil has a unique property which can enhance your mind, your body, and your spirit.

Chapter Three: Aromatherapy's Flexibility

Perhaps one of the most exciting aspects of aromatherapy is the fact that these oils are not limited to something you mix in your bath or pay for with a professional massage. You can integrate essential oils based on your needs at any given time. You can add oils to reusable aromatherapy candle holders. You can mix them into your bath or add them to your food. You can create homemade masks to revive your skin which include adding a few drops of your favorite oil. You can keep a jar of your favorite oils on hand so that when the moment of stress arrives you can quickly dab them under your tongue, on your skin or inhale them through your nose. The flexibility afforded by this historic method of stress reduction in weight loss is perhaps one of it's best features. You can purchase a handful of oils recommended for stress relief and weight loss, and after testing them out to determine which ones you aligned with the best, you can invest in larger quantities of those and mix them in with your lotions, shower gels, massages, drinks, food and much more. The creativity is truly in your hands. You can even use aromatherapy in your meditation at home.

Herbology

For the last few thousand years, practitioners of traditional proven and pain-free Chinese medicinal cures have utilized an array of herbs for the healing properties they possess. There are well over three hundred therapeutic herbs that have been safely and effectively used throughout the centuries. Practitioners often find herbs to use in conjunction with acupuncture and/or other treatments. Different herbal formulas are designed by practitioners based on the individual needs of the patient. Even if you have the same diagnosis as another patient, it is highly unlikely that you will receive the same prescription of herbs.

Qigong

Qigong is a holistic system of exercise and meditation which is passed down from generations in China. It literally translates to "working with one's life energy". It is an evolving practice that includes breathing techniques, meditation, self-massage, movement, and healing postures. The goal of it is to eliminate bad *Qi* and develop good *Qi* in a manner that becomes as second nature as breathing. You can integrate this form of healing into aromatherapy by having essential oils burning in the form of candles while you meditate.

Chapter Four: Aromatherapy and Sleep

Aromatherapy improves your sleep. Sleep can actually give you healthier skin. Your body needs sleep in order to promote healthy skin but you also need to be cautious about which type of bedding you use in order to protect your face from wrinkles over time.

Sleep is important to ensuring you have natural, healthy, beautiful younger looking skin. When you sleep you are giving your body a chance to repair itself. This means that it repairs everything at a cellular level. If you miss sleep regularly it can increase your risk of bad skin because you deprive your body of the opportunity to repair anything that is broken.

There are two states in the nervous system which must remain in balance. The first state is the sympathetic system which takes control when you are awake. During this state the majority of your blood flow goes to the core of your body. When you sleep you go into the parasympathetic nervous system. This system takes control and shifts the majority of the blood flow in your body to the skin. When you sleep your skin is also no longer prone to attacks from elements in the air. In the parasympathetic state your body and your cells are all more relaxed. This improves circulation and the flow of oxygen to your skin. During this phase your skin gets internal attention and repairs, the same as a business owner would make repairs to their office at night when the staff are away. The receptors in your body come to life. These receptors are inside your blood vessels and they take the amino acid molecules that your body needs to create more collagen and drain any toxins from your skin.

If you do not get enough sleep your skin does not have a chance to repair itself or restore the collagen it needs. One example of this is if you have excess fluid near your skin and you do not get enough sleep then that fluid will not be transported to your bladder for excretion. Instead it will leave you skin looking puffy. Why is this? Because in the parasympathetic state your kidneys are more active and they remove excess fluid from your circulatory system down to your bladder. This shows up most around your eyes because that area of skin has the least amount of fat and therefore the water your skin retains is more evident here. This is why you may see dark circles.

And when you sleep there are different fabrics which are best. There are ups and downs to each fabric. Satin sheets for example are actually considered one of the best materials you can have for your skin. They are soothing to your skin. They also allow you to sleep better as you lay in the softness. The fabric enables your skin to maintain the natural moisture it has as well. Cotton sheets may be comfortable, but they will absorb the majority of your skins natural moisture which can leave it dry and damaged over time. Satin bedding will also prevent wrinkles on your face so that you wake up more refreshed, and with naturally healthy and beautifully young looking skin. Because satin is so soft there is hardly any friction when you sleep which ensures your skin and your hair are well taken care of while you sleep without the risk of snagging and tangling or breaking.

Silk sheets are wrinkle free naturally which encourages your skin to slide across them when you sleep. There are also amino acids in silk sheets that help promote good skin and reduce the risk of premature wrinkles. Silk sheets are made from the cocoons of silk worms which mean they contain natural substances that repel things like mold and dust mites.

Cotton sheets are breathable but they take away the natural moisture from your skin. But if you are prone to acne or oily skin then cotton is a fabric that reduces the likelihood of sweating while you sleep. This is important because when you sweat during sleep it collects on your pillow and in your sheets and then comes into contact with your skin all night long. This can irritate those who suffer from acne and lead to further spots or irregular skin tones.

Bamboo sheets are much the same as cotton sheets but they have antibacterial properties which are non-irritating and hypoallergenic making them perfect for those who suffer from sensitive skin or acne.

Chapter Five: Top Aromatherapy Extracts

Top Aromatherapy Extracts

The evening primrose flower, or *Oenothera,* is bright yellow and produces small blooms that open at dusk. The oil extracted from the seeds are very effective in moisturizing dry skin and eradicating the dark circles under your eyes. Long utilized by Native Americans to treat wounds, bruises, burns and other skin problems, the plant originated in Central America and over time, extended its gifts to North and South America.

Since the 1930s, primrose oil has been utilized as a skin care supplement and as an anti-inflammatory. The combination of omega six fatty acids, gamma-linolenic acid and linolenic acid, proves astonishing in maintaining healthy bones, skin, and hair. This essential oil, taken either in capsule form or applied topically, is an integral part of a daily skin regimen. There are mixed reviews of the supplement's ability to ease eczema, but it overall it creates smoother, softer, and more supple skin.

In addition to the benefits of preserving a vibrant complexion, primrose oil has been found effective in combating inflammatory diseases such as dermatitis, rheumatoid arthritis, and diabetic retinopathy (a complication of diabetes that causes damage to the retina and may lead to blindness). Occasionally mild side effects such as nausea and headaches may occur, and primrose oil should not be taken if one is using a blood thinning or anticoagulant medication, so one should consult a physician before use.

Co-enzyme Q10, or ubiquinol, is a vitamin-like substance that is produced from a protein in our bodies and from our food intake. Its main function is to convert food into energy and therefore it is highly concentrated in the organs that require the most energy: the heart, liver, and kidneys. It also functions as an antioxidant, by preventing the oxidation of lipids in the body – key in promoting and maintaining collagen in our skin and keeping us fresh and radiant looking. The levels of co-enzyme Q10 in our bodies peaks in our twenties, and then declines steadily thereafter. Dietary imbalances, stress and smoking further deplete the concentration levels. Since the enzyme's purpose is the creation of energy, it follows that by compensating for the diminution of co-enzyme Q10, one can expect to see benefits such as increased energy, greater vitality, and a renewed sense of youthfulness and zest for life. Healthy heart function in particular demands a lot of energy, and with the natural depletion of this enzyme in our bodies, the heart is more susceptible to diseases and weakening. By taking this supplement, you can keep your heart healthy and sound well into old age. As co-enzyme Q10 also functions as an antioxidant, it targets and rids the body of free radicals, the waste products of cell metabolism, and minimizes the harmful effects of exposure to toxins such as cigarette smoke and pollution. The buildup of free radicals is responsible for the breakdown of cells and tissues in our bodies, and is injurious to the collagen in our skin. These free radicals are a major contributor to the adverse effects of aging and to health problems such as cardiovascular disease and cancer. Antioxidants such as co-enzyme Q10 eliminate these free radicals, thus preventing and diminishing the negative effects of aging, as well as stimulating skin repair and regeneration.

If you want to decrease the effects of daily stress and alleviate the signs of aging, take magnesium supplements. Magnesium is essential for energy production, muscle relaxation and calcium metabolism; indeed, calcium supplements need to be accompanied by magnesium for proper absorption and utilization in the bones and teeth. It is, apparently, the most underrated and remarkable mineral, though its benefits are miraculous.

The declining levels of nutrition in our genetically modified, processed and packaged food, not to mention the increasing levels of stress that so many of us are subject to, combine to render nearly everyone deficient in magnesium. This increases the risk for numerous health problems.

Magnesium is also an amazing antidote for pain, and is crucial in assuaging symptoms of stress circumventing the potential of age related disease. It is not enough to simply lather on creams and potions as we age. It is vital to take proactive measures to prevent illness and disease. Magnesium to the rescue! Magnesium diminishes muscle cramps and tension (take a bath in Epsom salts to relieve the soreness in your limbs), it lowers the risk of heart disease, reduces blood pressure, and significantly lowers the risk for sudden cardiac death. It is also widely beneficial for combating the visible signs of aging.

You can take 200 milligram capsules of magnesium twice daily, to ease aches, pains, headaches, and to help you sleep soundly and wake up feeling rested. Proper levels of magnesium counteract the effects of chronic stress, for stress will deplete magnesium.

In addition, magnesium is a regenerative mineral and prevents the calcification of organs and tissues that occurs during the aging process. Specifically, it keeps the skin rejuvenated and smooth looking, fighting dryness and wrinkles.

More and more people are moving away from pharmaceutical remedies to improve and maintain health and towards a more holistic, natural way - and taking chromium and zinc as a colloidal mineral supplement is one of the ways you can choose to maintain your health naturally. Colloidal mineral supplements are easier for the body to metabolize as they are suspended in water. Many capsule based supplements are not utilized within the body to their full potential. Colloidal mixtures solve that problem and are a safe and pure source of minerals. Colloidal chromium and zinc supplements are important to consider taking as they are not produced naturally by our bodies and are not included in most contemporary diets.

Chromium and zinc are among nine trace minerals required by the body in small amounts for general health and wellbeing, and are effective for fighting the aging process. They are known for their antioxidant effects, which increase the skin's vitality and battle the degenerative effects of free radicals in the body's cells and tissues, which is the number one factor in the detrimental effects of aging.

Chromium is essential in metabolism and the regulation of blood glucose levels, and it is especially beneficial for diabetics. You can take chromium to keep your weight controlled and boost energy. Zinc is effective in treating acne, supporting the immune system, and in the formation of healthy bones. Zinc also aids in the elimination of free radicals and encourages collagen production.

Chapter Six: Food and Stress

There are natural remedies to be found which will calm and relax you when you are stressed. Consider integrating the following natural remedies in some fashion such; in tea, baths or candles.

- Kava root

- Passionflower herb

- Lemon balm

- Lavender

- St. John's Wort

- Valerian

- Motherwort

- Skullcap

- Licorice root

- Chamomile

- Oat straw

Lemon

Lemon is another great medicinal plant. It is actually from India and was brought over to America during the second voyage by Columbus. Lemon trees are sharp and have thick spines. The leaves are about 5cm long and the tree has white flowers. The fruit is round and oval shaped with small white seeds. Lemon has a lot of great benefits to ensure you look and feel younger at the turning point of life. It has:

· Essential oils

· Vitamin C

· Carotenoids

· Sugar

· Citric acid

It is great for therapeutic indications and pharmacological activity. In fact it has a lot of antibacterial and decongestant properties. It can also be used for healing and as a re-mineralizing agent or diuretic. It can help with:

· Fevers

· Flues

· Hemorrhoids

· Hypertension

· Diarrhea

- Obesity

- Common colds

Turmeric

Turmeric is a perennial herb that has aromatic rhizomes. It is used mostly as seasoning in curries but also has anticancer properties. It is therapeutic and can be used to prevent:

- Hepatitis

- Cholecystitis

- Atherosclerosis

- Thrombosis

Ginger

Ginger is great for keeping yourself healthy during the turning point of your life. It is often used in treatment against ovarian cancer and colon cancer. It can be used to treat morning sickness too. It offers migraine relief because it stops prostaglandins from causing inflammation in your blood vessels. It can be used to fight cold and flu symptoms and has positive effects on the digestive tract. Ginger naturally treats heartburn and can be consumed in tea to treat menstrual cramps.

Mint

Mint has many medicinal properties. It is an herb that is used for its essential oils and its caffeic acid. It can be used as an antibacterial and antiseptic as well as an anti-inflammatory. It is also used as an anti fungal and a choleretic. Therapeutically it is used to treat:

- Diarrhea

- Dermatitis

- Flatulence

- Asthma

- Asthenia

- Anorexia

Sugar

If you consume too much sugar over a long period of time it can lead to wrinkles and dull skin. The reason for this is premature aging in your body, a process called gycation. The process causes the sugar in your bloodstream to attach to proteins which create harmful molecules. The harmful molecules damage the proteins in your naturally healthy and beautifully young looking skin, particularly the elastin fibers and the collagen. Both of these keep your skin elastic and supple. Because collagen is the most popular protein in your body, as soon as it becomes damaged it leads to sagging skin.

These effects can start at the age of 35 and increase in an incredibly fast fashion! Therefore you should limit the amount of sugar you consume not just for the sake of your waist, but for your skin!

There are certain foods which you can consume to fight off sun damage and wrinkles. You can boost your natural defence against skin cancer and keep your skin looking naturally healthy and beautifully young by eating these foods:

#1: Strawberries

Eating one cup of strawberries per day will give your body the amount of vitamin C it requires to fight off wrinkles and the signs of ageing related to dry skin.

#2: Tomatoes:

Tomatoes are red. Everyone knows that. But not everyone knows why. They are red because of lycopene. This is a cartenoid and it can help keep your skin silky smooth. By consuming more tomatoes you can also protect your skin from sunburn.

#3: Tofu

This is a soy food which will preserve firm skin because of the isoflavones. It reduces wrinkles in people exposed to the sun and gives you smoother skin. The reason being, it prevents collagen breakdown.

#4: Tuna

Tuna has a nice amount of omega-3 fatty acids which prevent cancer and preserve collagen in your skin. This keeps your skin healthy and younger. It also prevents skin cancer because it reduces inflammation which promotes the growth of tumours.

#5: Coffee

Drinking one cup of coffee each day will reduce the risk of developing skin cancer by ten percent. But decaf does not offer the same benefits.

Hydrating foods

While drinking plenty of water is important, there are many fruits and vegetables that provide hydration. Cucumbers contain ninety six percent water, pineapple is comprised of ninety five percent water, watermelon at ninety four percent, grapefruit contains ninety percent, and blueberries are ninety five percent. Melon is ninety two percent water, celery is ninety six percent, tomatoes are ninety four percent and romaine lettuce is ninety five percent water.

Fabulous fruit

Cherries will calm your nervous system. Grapes will relax your blood vessels. Peaches have a high content of potassium and iron as well as fluoride. Apples will help to protect your body and develop resistance to infections. Watermelon can help control your heart rate. Oranges will maintain great vision and skin. Strawberries can fight against aging and cancer. Bananas give you energy. Pineapples help to fight arthritis. Blueberries protect your heart. Kiwis will increase bone mass and mangoes will protect against several forms of cancer.

Calcium:

Calcium is present in dairy products as well as broccoli, salmon and kale. The daily recommendation is 1000 mg. As a point of reference 8 ounces of non-fat milk is equal to 299 mg. Calcium supports strong bones, teeth, and muscle function. It also sustains healthy heart rhythm and prevents high blood pressure.

Fiber:

Fiber can be found in grains as well as beans and produce. The daily recommended dose is 25-35 grams. As a point of reference one baked potato has 3.8 grams. It will lower cholesterol and improve digestion. It will also reduce the risk of heart disease.

Magnesium:

Magnesium is prevalent in nuts as well as peas and beans. It is also present in whole grains and spinach. The daily recommended amount of magnesium is 500 mg. As a point of reference one ounce of almonds equals 80 mg. Magnesium deficiencies are linked to diabetes as well as osteoporosis, high blood pressure, and muscle cramps.

Potassium:

You can find potassium in avocados and potatoes. It is also present in bananas, milk and sweet potatoes. It is recommended that you get 4.6 grams daily. As a point of reference one banana is equal to . 4 grams. Potassium is beneficial in reducing high blood pressure, while it promotes fertility and improves muscle and nerve function.

Vitamin A:

It can be found in sweet potatoes and carrots as well as spinach and broccoli. The daily recommended amount of vitamin A is 5000 IU. Ten baby carrots are equal to 13800 IU which is 276% of your daily value. Vitamin A supports good vision and tissue growth, and is of great benefit to a healthy immune system.

Vitamin C:

Vitamin C is found in bell peppers and leafy greens. It can also be found in strawberries and oranges as well as kiwis. The daily recommended dose of Vitamin C is 80 mg. As a point of reference ½ strawberry is equal to 49 mg. Vitamin C supports immunity first and foremost. It also boosts the growth of bones and tissue while protecting your cells from free radicals.

Vitamin D:

Vitamin D is found in sunlight, salmon and mushrooms. It is also present in liver, cheese and fortified cereal. The daily recommended dose of Vitamin D is 400 IU. As a point of reference three ounces of salmon contains 447 IU which is 112% of your daily value. It supports healthy bones as well as muscle nerve fibers and the immune system.

Chapter Seven: Scientific Studies

Today aromatherapy is used in conjunction with certain pharmaceutical treatments. In order to establish the scientific evidence for the effectiveness of these treatments double blind and placebo controlled trials must take place.

It should be noted that these studies do not account for the principle within Western medicine that specific aromatherapy regimes and treatments must be catered directly to individuals, and must be revisited regularly by a practitioner. They were, however, conducted in order to adhere to the requirements of Western practitioners who were unsatisfied with the concept of assigning specific herbal groupings with other components of Western medicine to treat the entire person inside and out, rather than a single syndrome. Nonetheless, the studies still show very positive results "proving" for Western practitioners that these methods are extremely effective. Please note, again, that these aromatherapy remedies MUST be prescribed by a practitioner and the preparation and consumption must be per their requirements exactly, the same as any other prescription.

Another study was conducted for the Kampo formula that mixed licorice with rhubarb in order to counter constipation, something that is often a side effect of stress and can lead to weight gain. A two week long study which was double blind, and placebo controlled, tested one hundred and thirty two people who were randomly assigned high doses of the herbal treatment, low doses of the herbal treatment, and a placebo. The results of this test indicate that the group receiving the higher dose experienced significant improvements compared to the placebo counterpart.

There was a double blind study conducted with two hundred patients who suffered from diabetes. It tested whether a traditional combination therapy was effective in fighting against diabetes. The results showed that using a traditional combination therapy produced the greatest benefits when it was used without pharmaceutical drugs and it was able to treat diabetes.

There is a popular topical ointment which is referred to as Tiger Balm, often used to treat tension headaches. It mixes camphor, clove oil, cajaput, and menthol. A study was conducted with fifty seven participants who applied it to their forehead and took Tylenol. The results showed that the Tiger Balm was much more effective than the placebo, and more rapid-acting than taking Tylenol.

In a review of twenty one studies which involved over three thousand patients, researchers were able to conclude that herbs were effective in treating illness, and also lacked the withdrawal symptoms traditionally associated with prescription medication. Other tests have generated positive results for the use of Chinese medicine to treat the symptoms of stress, psoriasis, acute pancreatitis, dementia, bi-polar syndrome, and weight loss.

Chapter Eight: Safety Tips

Perhaps one of the most important safety considerations is that each essential oil you use should be used in moderation, adhering to the recommended amounts based on whether you are burning, inhaling, ingesting, or mixing them. Nutrition and herbs have remained an important part of treatment protocols for thousands of years. They can extend the positive effects of other aspects of treatment such as acupuncture, particularly for people who might otherwise be subject to treatment multiple times each week. Herbal formulas are designed to target a specific problem by the healthcare practitioner. With aromatherapy the substances are taken from minerals and plants. They are combined into formulas which often include between eight and fifteen ingredients which work together.

When oils are prescribed by a practitioner, and the instructions from said practitioner adhered to, they are very safe. In fact, they are just as safe as the food you would consume each day. Many people do not realize that the herbs prescribed in most treatment regimens can be eaten as food. The preparation and frequency of consumption are responsible for the potency of the effects. If the wrong herb is taken, or the dosage is incorrect, it can be dangerous, which is why it is important to adhere to the instructions of your practitioner.

Some people are concerned with the risk of contamination, especially when it comes to herbs shipped from around the world and manufactured to all different standards. But a practitioner will ensure you are given the highest quality herbs, as they are known for adhering to strict quality control.

Herbal medications are supported by anecdotal evidence from practitioners and patients around the world and are applied to a myriad of conditions. Some herbs can help with digestive issues like Barrett's Oesophagus or oesophageal cancer. There are different herbal supplements that may be integrated into your treatment. Different teas and herbs are combined for different conditions and individuals.

One example is green tea. This is known for its high amount of polyphenols. It protects against the development of tumours because it suppresses cell proliferation or the changing of cells into cancer cells. This tea has a high dose of antioxidants as well, which helps to remove toxins from your body. Green tea will also stimulate the lower esophageal sphincter which is a muscle responsible for stopping your stomach acid from leaking into your esophagus and damaging the lining of your throat. Green tea can increase your blood pressure because of the caffeine levels but there are non-caffeinated versions available.

Licorice root is one famous herb that is now used throughout Eastern and Western medicine. It elevates the prostaglandin levels in your body which increases the formation of mucus. This can be used to treat things such as heart burn because it improves cellular health and coats the throat and esophagus with mucus, which prevents damage done by stomach acid sneaking back up. This herb may increase your blood pressure and will thin your blood. This is good if you have blood clots from stagnant *qi,* but it is important that you ensure you adhere to your practitioner's dosage and advice.

Oldenlandia diffusae is another herb that will reduce heat in your body and remove toxins. Chinese rhubarb is used by Chinese medicinal practitioners to clean your blood and remove toxins. Herbal Selaginella doerderleinii is used to prevent the new growth of tumours and slow tumour growth that has already started. Ginger tea will also increase the antioxidants in your body and improve the health of your digestive system. Panax ginseng is the most widely used herb in all of pain-free traditional Chinese medicine, because it boosts energy and enhances the immune system. Ginseng is broadly used in the treatment of cancer or immune system function.

One of the most highly regarded herbs proven in its effectiveness is ephedra. This is one of the most widely used herbs in proven and pain-free Aromatherapy cures, and is often used to induce sweating or treat asthma. But it is hardly ever used as a single agent. In America, western doctors often sell it as a form of herbal caffeine at truck stops or anywhere else that people want to get a "buzz". It is also poorly promoted as a means of weight loss.

Aconite is another popular herb proven in its pain-free effectiveness. It is a hot herb that is often found in traditional proven and pain-free Aromatherapy cures to help relieve severe cold diagnoses. In its raw form this herb is cardio toxic which is why it must be boiled for a minimum of one hour before it is used. It also has a narrow window in which its therapeutic value can be used. This is why it is so important that herb treatment plans prescribed by a practitioner are strictly followed.

Astragalus is promoted because of its ability to help build up the immune system or *qi* in a person. It can move the life energy from deep levels in the body to the surface of the body. Cinnabar is used in proven and pain-free Aromatherapy cures as a sedative.

When you prepare herbal tea you should place the prescribed amount of the tea leaves into boiling water and let them sit for five minutes. Once this is done you should remove the tea from heat and allow it to steep for another fifteen minutes. Once you have done this you can consume the tea at cool or warm temperatures. If the taste is unpleasant you can add a teaspoon of honey to help make it a bit sweeter.

With any herb it is important that you look for fresh herbs that have been newly dried. You can shop at select specialty herbal stores that have a high turnover rate. This ensures the herbs do not sit on the shelf for a long time. You can speak with your practitioner about the best places to buy herbs.

Decoctions

The majority of Aromatherapy oils must be prepared through decoction. This means that you boil the herbs in water in order to extract the concentration and ensure potency and quick effects. The proper preparation may be time consuming, but the therapeutic benefits are well worth it.

Granulated Extracts

If you do not have to deal with decoctions then you can opt for granulated extracts. This form of herbal treatment offers comparable results. These herbs are freeze dried with corn starch or potato starch to offer quick preparation. They can be mixed with boiling water to dissolve the granules and then consumed.

BONUS DIY RECIPIE MATERIAL TO FOLLOW...

Essential Oil Recipes for Skin Care and Stress Relief

1. Stress Relieving Roll On

Ingredients:

1 drop geranium oil

2 drops Roman chamomile oil

3 drops Bergaptene-free bergamot oil

4 drops lavender oil

2 teaspoons "for skin care" grapeseed oil

Method:

Place grapeseed oil in a dark glass rollerball bottle using a small funnel. Add all your essential oils and shake gently to mix.

TO USE: Roll on neck and wrists.

2. Aromatherapy Stress Reduction Inhaler

Ingredients:

1 teaspoon coarse sea salt

1 drop chamomile oil

1 drop Rose Geranium oil

4 drops orange oil

4 drops lavender oil

10 drops bergamot oil

Method:

Place salt in a small dark glass. Add all the essential oils. Gently shake to combine.

TO USE: Have three deep, long, and slow breaths of aroma. Rest in a while. Have 3 deep breaths again. Rest and have the final 3 deep breaths with the aroma.

3.Calming Bath Oil

Ingredients:

2 drops cedarwood oil

12 drops lavender oil

30 drops sandalwood oil

4fl oz jojoba oil

Method:

Gently place all your essential oils in a PET plastic bottle. Shake to combine and store it in a dark, cool place.

TO USE: Place 1 tablespoon into your bath after you have complet-ed running the water.

4. Relaxing Massage Oil

Ingredients:

¼ cup jojoba oil

1 drop vetiver oil

2 drops clary sage oil

3 drops marjoram oil

12 drops orange oil

12 drops lavender oil

Method:

Place all your essential oils in a dark glass. Gently shake and leave it for at least 24 hours before using. Store it in a dark and cool place. This will last up to 3 months.

5. Sleep Well Linen Spray

Ingredients:

2 ounces distilled water

20 drops lavender oil

1 teaspoon witch hazel

Method:

Place lavender oil in a glass bottle with a spray cap. Add witch hazel and distilled water. Shake well to combine.

TO USE: Spray it on your clean linen, pillows, or clothes before sleeping.

6.So Relaxing Bath Salts

Ingredients:

1 cup Epsom salts

5 drops copaiba oil

10 drops PanAway oil

Method:

Place Epsom salts in a glass bowl along with your essential oils. Using a metal spoon, mix it until well combined. Transfer it in an 8 oz glass pot and cover tightly.

TO USE: Scoop ¼ - ½ cup and place into a warm bath.

7.Sleep Potion

Ingredients:

2 oz Ancient Minerals magnesium oil

5 drops cedarwood oil

5 drops tangerine oil

10 drops lavender oil

Method:

Place your Ancient Minerals magnesium oil in a spray bottle along with the essential oils. Shake it well to combine.

TO USE: Rub it in your feet about 20 minutes before sleeping.

8.Calming Bubble Bath

Ingredients:

1 teaspoon chamomile oil

1 teaspoon pure vanilla extract

¼ cup pure vegetable glycerin

1 cup mild liquid body soap

Method:

Place all ingredients in a plastic bottle and shake very gently to combine.

TO USE: Place ½ cup under running water.

9.Anxiety Relief Lavender Rub

Ingredients:

1 teaspoon fractionated almond oil

3 drops lavender oil

Method:

Place almond oil in your palm. Add lavender oil and blend them together.

TO USE: Rub it onto your neck or bottoms of feet just before sleeping.

10.Stress Relief Room Mist

Ingredients:

2 drops rose oil

4 drops Ylang Ylang oil

14 drops bergamot oil

20 drops lime oil

4 oz. clean spray bottle with a fine mist setting

3 fl. ounces distilled water

Method:

Place distilled water in your 4 oz spray bottle. Add essential oil. Shake it to combine.

To Use: Shake bottle before each use. Lightly mist your room. Make sure mist will not fall into open beverages and onto furniture.

11. Sleep Well Shower Steamer

Ingredients:

30 drops lavender oil

12 drops Frankincense oil

12 drops sandalwood oil

2 drops Vetiver oil

2 drops Geranium oil

2 cups baking soda

1 cup citric acid

A spray bottle of witch hazel

Method:

Strain citric acid and baking soda through a fine sieve. Press out any lumps. Mix citric acid and baking soda together. Add your essential oils, stirring it as you go to avoid any clumps. Mist witch hazel over your mixture with just the amount necessary to moisten and bind together. Stir it briskly with a fork. Squeeze, spray, and stir until clump will hold its shape. Press it very firmly into molds. Leave it for 30 minutes or so. Unmold and allow them to sit undisturbed overnight to fully dry up. Lightly cover using a cling wrap.

Wrap them with parchment paper and place in a container and seal tightly.

12. Peppermint Bath

Ingredients:

½ cup Baking soda

10 drops peppermint oil

Handful of Epsom salts

Method:

While drawing your hot bath, add all the ingredients and soak for about 20 minutes. Perform this procedure once a week. For 5 minutes, rinse off with a cool shower.

13. Hydrating Lavender Soap Bar

Ingredients:

Soap Base

3 drops Vitamin E

25 drops lavender oil

Method:

Melt soap base in a glass bowl in a saucepan with water. Turn off heat and allow it to cool a little bit. Stir in vitamin E and lavender oil. Mix well to combine. Pour mixture into a soap mold and allow to cool completely. Pop it out and keep in a room temperature place.

14. Nourishing Lotion

Ingredients:

20 drops each of myrrh and frankincense oil

¼ cup each of olive oil and coconut oil

¼ cup each of Beeswax and shea butter

2 tablespoons Vitamin E

BPA free plastic lotion dispenser bottles

Method:

Melt together beeswax, shea butter, olive oil, and coconut oil in a glass bowl in a saucepan with water until mixed well. Allow it to cool slightly and place put in your refrigerator until firm, about an hour. Whip mixture with a hand mixer until fluffy. Mix in vitamin E and essential oils. Transfer it in a BPA-free plastic lotion dispenser bottle and store in cool place.

15. Cellulite Scrub

Ingredients:

1 cup organic ground coffee

½ cup olive oil

10 drops grapefruit oil

5 drops Cypress oil

Method:

Mix coffee and olive oil in a large glass bowl using a metal spoon. Stir in essential oils. Transfer mixture in a glass pot and seal tightly. Store it in a cool and dark place.

TO USE: Gently rub mixture into body parts with cellulites for a few minutes, then rinse.

16.Shaving Cream

Ingredients:

3 tablespoons olive oil

1 teaspoon Castile soap

1/3 cup each of coconut oil and shea butter

8 drops peppermint oil

Method:

Melt coconut oil and shea butter in a double boiler over low heat. Remove from heat and transfer in a glass bowl. Stir in olive oil and allow it to cool slightly. Stir in Castile soap along with the peppermint oil. Chill it in your refrigerator until it begins to firm, about an hour. Whip it using an immersion blender until fluffy. Transfer solution in a glass pot and seal tightly. Store it in a dark and cool place.

17. Shaving Gel

Ingredients:

7 drops each of lemongrass oil and grapefruit oil

¼ cup olive oil

¾ cup aloe vera gel

Method:

Pour aloe vera gel into a pump bottle using a small funnel. Add olive oil along with the essential oils. Seal bottle tightly and shake well to combine. Store it in a cool and dark place.

18. Hydrating After Shave

Ingredients:

10 drops each of orange and sandalwood oil

2 tablespoons jojoba oil

½ cup each of aloe vera gel and witch hazel

1 teaspoon Vitamin E oil

Method:

Place aloe vera gel in a pump bottle using a small funnel. Add Vitamin E oil, jojoba oil, and witch hazel. Lastly, add the essential oils and seal bottle. Shake it well and store in a cool and dark place.

19. Stretch Mark Reducing Rub

Ingredients:

5 drops each of geranium and lavender oil

¼ cup olive oil

½ cup each of cocoa butter and shea butter

1 tablespoon Vitamin E oil

Method:

Melt coconut oil, shea and cocoa butter in a double boiler over low heat. Remove from heat and transfer melted oil in a glass bowl. Allow it to cool slightly. Stir in Vitamin E oil along with the essential oils. Chill in your refrigerator until it begins to firm, about an hour. Whip it using an immersion blender and then place in a glass pot. Seal tightly and store in a dark and cool place.

TO USE: Apply it daily into your body parts with stretch marks.

20. Foot Rub

Ingredients:

10 drops Thieves oil

10 drops oregano oil

20 drops extra virgin olive oil

Method:

Place all ingredients in a roll-on bottle. Seal tightly.

TO USE: Apply it to the bottom of your feet when needed.

21.Lotion Bars

Ingredients:

25 drops Melrose oil

25 drops lavender oil

¼ cup shea butter

¼ cup coconut oil

¼ cup grated beeswax, firmly packed

Method:

Melt coconut oil, shea butter, and beeswax in a bowl set over simmering water in a saucepan. Take it off from heat. Stir in essential oils and pour solution into a mold. Allow it to cool and firm. Unmold and store in an airtight container.

22.Facial Serum

Ingredients:

1 oz jojoba oil

2 drops Frankincense oil

2 drops sandalwood oil

1 drop rose oil

Method:

Place your essential oils along with the jojoba oil in a 1 oz amber bottle that is fitted with a glass dropper. Shake gently to combine.

23. Cooling Toner

Ingredients:

30 drops peppermint oil

¼ cup apple cider vinegar

¾ cup filtered water

Method:

Place all ingredients in a glass bottle. Shake it gently to combine and store in your refrigerator.

TO USE: Mist your face lightly especially after your face cleansing.

24. Body Butter

Ingredients:

30 drops peppermint oil

½ cup coconut oil

½ cup cocoa butter

Method:

Place cocoa butter and coconut oil in a mixing bowl. Add the peppermint oil. Whip mixture using a hand mixer until it is airy and perfectly whipped. Transfer in a glass container and store in a cool and dry place.

25.Lemon Foaming Hand Soap

Ingredients:

1/8 teaspoon lemon essential oil

2/3 cup filtered water

1/3 cup liquid unscented Castile soap

Method:

Stir Castile soap in a jar along with your essential. Add water. Seal tightly and shake to mix.

26.Hand Sanitizer

Ingredients:

10 drops Thieves oil

¼ teaspoon Vitamin E oil

¼ cup aloe vera gel

2 tablespoon filtered water

Method:

Mix all ingredients and place in a small plastic bottle.

27.Lip Balm

Ingredients:

15 drops Lavender oil

5 drops Frankincense oil

2 tablespoons beeswax

2 tablespoons coconut oil

1 tablespoon sweet almond oil

1 tablespoon shea butter

½ teaspoon raw honey

Method:

Melt together honey, coconut oil, beeswax, and shea butter in a double boiler. Turn off heat and stir in your essential oils along with the sweet almond oil. Pour mixture right away into lip balm tubes. Allow it to set and seal tightly.

28. Foaming Facial Wash

Ingredients:

10 drops Ylang Ylang oil

5 drops Patchouli oil

4 drops lemongrass oil

2/3 cup filtered water

1/3 cup castile soap

½ teaspoon sweet almond oil

Method:

Place all ingredients into a foaming soap dispenser, leaving water behind. Swirl mixture to combine. Add water. Seal tightly and shake gently to combine.

29. Deodorant

Ingredients:

10 drops Purification oil

6 tablespoons arrowroot powder

3 tablespoons shea butter

2 tablespoons coconut oil

2 tablespoons Bentonite clay

1 tablespoon baking soda

Method:

Combine all dry ingredients in a bowl. Whip coconut oil and shea butter using a stand mixer until mixed well. Reduce speed to low while slowly adding your essential oil and 1/3 of dry ingredients. Mix it well and add another 1/3 of dry ingredients. Mix well and add the rest of dry ingredients. Take the mixture out. Roll it into a ball and press into an airtight glass jar. Store it in a cool and dry place.

30. Rosemary Shampoo

Ingredients:

15 drops rosemary oil

2 drops peppermint oil

½ cup filtered water

½ cup castile soap

Method:

Place castile soap in a flip top container. Add your essential oils along with the water. Shake it to incorporate.

31.Bug Repellent Spray

Ingredients:

8 drops Geranium oil

5 drops rosemary oil

5 drops lavender oil

2 drops Patchouli

1 ½ tablespoons Distilled water

1 teaspoon sweet almond oil

1 teaspoon Witch hazel

Method:

Place all ingredients in a spray bottle. Place the lid and shake well to combine. Careful not to spray in your mouth and eyes.

32.Itch Control Spray

Ingredients:

5 drops lavender oil

3 drops tea tree oil

2 drops Frankincense oil

Witch hazel

Method:

Place witch hazel to the shoulder of a 2 oz spray bottle. Add the rest of ingredients. Seal and shake well to combine.

33.Eczema Cream

Ingredients:

15 drops lavender oil

5 drops tea tree oil

¼ cup coconut oil

¼ cup shea butter

Method:

Place coconut oil and shea butter in a mason jar. Place it in a saucepan halfway full with simmering water. Allow butter and oil to melt. Take the Mason jar out the pan and allow it to cool slightly. Stir in essential oils and then place jar in your refrigerator to firm up. Whip oil on high using a mixer for a few minutes. Transfer cream in a small container and store inside your refrigerator.

TO USE: Apply generously to affected area of your skin.

34.Psoriasis Remedy

Ingredients:

Fractionated Coconut Oil

35 drops oregano oil

5 drops patchouli oil

Method:

Place essential oils in a 10 ml roller ball bottle. Add fractionated coconut oil to fill the bottle.

TO USE: Apply cream on affected areas twice a day.

35.Varicose Veins Massage Oil

Ingredients:

2 ounce jojoba oil

2 oz avocado oil

20 drops lemongrass oil

10 drops helichrysum oil

10 drops cypress oil

6 drops frankincense oil

6 drops rosemary oil

6 drops chamomile oil

1 teaspoon Vitamin E oil

Method:

Place all ingredients in a dark spray bottle. Seal and shake it gently to mix. Store in a cool place.

TO USE: Massage affected area with this oil for 2-3 times a day.

36. Facial Moisturizer

Ingredients:

16 drops Frankincense oil

8 drops tea tree oil

4 drops lavender oil

½ cup cocoa butter

½ cup coconut oil

Method:

Combine all ingredients and whip them together. Transfer in a plastic bottle. Seal and store in a dark place.

37. Cracked Foot Salve

Ingredients:

5 drops lavender oil

3 drops sandalwood oil

2 drops German chamomile oil

2 teaspoons Vitamin E

3 oz coconut oil

1 oz raw cocoa butter

1 oz avocado oil

1 oz beeswax

1 oz tamanu oil

Method:

Leaving behind the essential oils and Vitamin E, melt all ingredients in a bowl in a double boiler. Remove from heat and stir in essential oils and Vitamin E. Transfer mixture into a glass container and allow it to cool for at least 30 minutes.

Use It: Apply it to your feet just before sleeping time. Wear socks after applying.

38.Solid Perfume

Ingredients:

30 drops sandalwood oil

30 drops grapefruit oil

30 drops vanilla oil

25 drops bergamot oil

4 tablespoons jojoba oil

4 tablespoons grated, packed beeswax

Method:

Place beeswax in a glass bowl and melt in a double boiler on low heat. Stir in jojoba oil and remove from heat as soon as they are blended well. Allow it to cool slightly and stir in your essential oils. Gently pour solution into a mold and allow it to firm up. Unmold and place in a nice container. Seal and store in a cool place.

39. Vanilla Body Spray

Ingredients:

2 drops Ylang Ylang oil

¼ cup witch hazel with alcohol

18 drops vanilla oleoresin

Method:

Combine all the ingredients. Transfer in a glass spray bottle and store in a cool and dark place.

TO USE: Shake it well before using. Apply it to your skin or clothes.

40. Lemon Body Scrub

Ingredients:

20 drops lemon essential oil

1 cup cane sugar

2 tablespoons lemon zest

¼ cup olive oil, melted

¼ cup of coconut oil

Method:

Combine melted coconut oil with olive oil, lemon oil, zest, and sugar. Mix well and place in a jar.

TO USE: Apply on your body generously.

41.Lavender Hair Pomade

Ingredients:

¼ teaspoon lavender oil

2 oz jojoba oil

1.5 oz shea butter

1 oz organic beeswax

Method:

Place beeswax in bowl and melt in a double boiler over low heat. Stir in shea butter until melted. Stir in jojoba oil. Transfer mixture in a container and allow it to cool slightly. Stir in your essential oil.

TO USE: Take a small amount of pomade between your fingertips. Rub it until there are no lumps. Work it through your hair.

42.Chamomile Hair Gel

Ingredients:

½ teaspoon gelatin

½ cup very warm purified water

5 drops chamomile oil

Method:

Dissolve your gelatin in ½ cup of very warm purified water. Remove from heat and allow it to cool slightly. Stir in essential oil. Transfer inn a container with lid and store in your fridge for 1-2 weeks.

43.Lip Tint

Ingredients:

4 drops peppermint oil

1 drop lemon oil

1 drop vanilla oil

2 tablespoons coconut oil

1 tablespoon shea butter

1 tablespoon beeswax

½ teaspoon rose mica powder

Method:

Melt together beeswax, coconut oil, and shee butter in a glass in double boiler. Remove from heat and allow it to cool slightly. Stir in your essential oils and rose mica powder. Transfer mixture into lip chap containers and allow it to cool completely.

44. Blackheads Face Scrub

Ingredients:

1 drop frankincense oil

1 drop lavender oil

1 drop geranium oil

1 tablespoon baking soda

½ tablespoon raw Manuka honey

Method:

Combine baking soda and honey to create paste. Stir in your essential oils.

TO USE: Take a warm washcloth and place over your face. Allow it to stay on your skin for a few minutes. Take your scrub and rub it in a circular motion on your skin for 4-5 minutes. Rinse face off with warm water.

45. Avocado Face Mask for Dry Skin

Ingredients:

3 drops Cedarwood oil

½ avocado, mashed

1 tablespoon aloe vera gel

1 tablespoon raw honey

Method:

Mix all ingredients in a bowl.

TO USE: Apply it all over your face and allow to sit for about 15-20 minutes. Rinse face with warm water.

46. Moisturizing Lotion

Ingredients:

15 drops lavender oil

5 drops rosemary oil

3 drops tea tree oil

3 drops carrot seed oil

2 tablespoons avocado oil

½ cup shea butter

Method:

Melt shea butter in a small pan over low heat. Stir in avocado oil. Remove from heat and place in a bowl. Allow it to cool slightly and place in your freezer for 15-20 minutes. Stir in the essential oils along with the carrot seed oil. Whip mixture for a minute. Transfer into a jar.

47.Anti-Aging Face Cream

Ingredients:

¼ teaspoon Rose hip seed oil

1 oz almond oil

1 oz coconut oil

1 packet organic green tea

.25 oz bees wax, grated

Method:

Melt together oil and wax in a double boiler. Stir in tea and allow it to warm for 15 minutes. Strain mixture through a fine mesh sieve directly into a bowl. Whip mixture using a hand mixer until creamy and transfer in a clean bottle. Store in a cool and dark place.

48.Face Wrinkle Cream

Ingredients:

3 drops lavender oil

1 drop carrot seed oil

¼ cup green tea

1 tablespoon rosehip seed oil

1 tablespoon sweet almond oil

1 teaspoon emulsifying wax

¼ teaspoon Vitamin E

1/8 teaspoon Neo Defend

Method:

Brew 1 cup green tea. Prepare 2 sauce pans and fill half way with water. Put a glass bowl with a spout to each pan. Turn heat to medium. To the one pot, place rosehip seed oil, wax, sweet almond oil, and Vitamin E oil. To the other pot, place NeoDefend and green tea respectively. Heat mixtures until wax has melted completely. Both mixture should reach 130 degrees. Combine both of them and mix using a hand blender. Work periodically for an hour. Stir in essential oils and carefully pour into prepared containers.

TO USE: This can be used during morning and night and works great under your make up. Careful not to pull or push on your skin.

49. Anti-Aging Eye Cream

Ingredients:

10 drops Frankincense oil

8 Vitamin E capsules

½ cup organic coconut oil, melted

Method:

Place melted oil in your container. Carefully poke each holes of Vitamin E capsules and squeeze liquid into container. Add essential oil. Place in your refrigerator for about 40-45 minutes.

TO USE: During the night, dab a small amount under your eyes.

50.Feminine Wash

Ingredients:

6 drops lavender oil

3 teaspoons almond oil

½ cup rose water

½ cup alcohol free witch hazel

1 teaspoon unscented castile soap

Method:

Place all the ingredients in a pump dispenser and swirl it to blend.